Alzheimer's and Dementia Awareness

Memory Loss, Care, and Support

Phillip J. Richmond

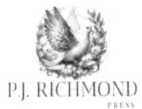

P.J. RICHMOND
PRESS

© 2024 by Phillip J. Richmond.

All rights reserved.

No part of this book may be reproduced, distributed, or transmitted in any form or by any means, including photocopying, recording, or other electronic or mechanical methods, without the prior written permission of the author, except in the case of brief quotations embodied in critical reviews and certain other noncommercial uses permitted by law. The author has made every effort to ensure the accuracy of the information in this book, but does not assume any responsibility for errors, omissions, or contrary interpretations of the subject matter herein. This book is provided "as is" without warranty of any kind, either expressed or implied. The author does not endorse or recommend any products, services, or websites that may be mentioned or referenced in this book.

For permission requests, write to the author at
philliprichmond92@gmail.com

Dedication

To those who navigate the foggy paths of memory loss,
To the caregivers who walk beside them with unwavering support,
And to the relentless spirit of hope that guides us all
Towards understanding, care, and a future free from Alzheimer's and dementia.

This book is dedicated to you.

More Books By Phillip J. Richmond

Overcoming Trauma From Rape
How to Stop Masturbation
Breaking Free
The Problem of Grief
How to Be A Better Partner
Quick Wit, Confident Speech
Arthritis Pain Relief
Heart Disease Prevention
Cancer Survival Guide

FACTS:

While age is the primary risk factor for Alzheimer's disease and dementia, other factors can also contribute to the development of these conditions. These include genetics, family history, cardiovascular health, traumatic brain injury, and lifestyle factors such as diet, exercise, and cognitive activity.

Contents

Dedication 3
How to Use This Book 7
Chapter 1: Understanding Alzheimer's and Dementia 9
    Defining Alzheimer's and Dementia 9
    The Science of Memory Loss 10
    Early Signs and Symptoms 11
    Diagnosis and Stages 13
Chapter 2: The Emotional Impact 17
    Living with a Diagnosis 17
    Emotional Reactions and Support 18
    The Caregiver's Role 20
    Coping Strategies for Families 21
Chapter 3: Medical Care and Management 25
    Treatment Options 25
    Managing Daily Life 27
    Safety Measures 28
    Future Therapies and Research 30
    Chapter 4: Legal and Financial Planning 35

    Preparing for the Future...35
    Legal Documents and Rights... 37
    Financial Strategies and Assistance......................................39

Chapter 5: Caregiving Essentials..42
    The Basics of Caregiving.. 42
    Creating a Supportive Environment...................................... 43
    Daily Routine and Activities... 45
    Respite Care and Support Groups.. 46

Chapter 6: Advance Care Considerations......................... 49
    Long-Term Care Options.. 49
    Palliative and End-of-Life Care...51
    Grief and Bereavement.. 52

Chapter 7: Building Awareness and Advocacy....................57
    Raise Public Awareness..57
    Advocacy and Policy Change.. 58
    Community Resources and Support....................................60

Glossary of Terms... 65
My Note..73
Special Bonus..81

How to Use This Book

Welcome to "Alzheimer's and Dementia Awareness: Memory Loss, Care, and Support." This book is a comprehensive guide designed to empower readers with knowledge, practical advice, and emotional support. Whether you are a caregiver, a healthcare professional, or someone who wants to learn more about these conditions, this book aims to be an invaluable resource.

Each chapter of this book focuses on a different aspect of Alzheimer's and dementia. The chapters are structured to take you on a journey from understanding the basics to mastering the complexities of care and support. You can read the book from start to finish or use the table of contents to find specific information relevant to your needs.

Throughout the book, you'll find interactive elements such as checklists, worksheets, and reflection questions. These tools are designed to help you apply the information to your personal situation, making the book a dynamic resource that grows with you.

Medical terms and concepts can be challenging, so I've included a glossary of terms and appendices with additional resources. These sections will help you clarify terminology and provide further reading and contacts for support.

This book can also serve as a discussion starter. Use it to facilitate conversations with family members, healthcare teams, or support groups. Sharing experiences and knowledge is a powerful way to build a community of care.

The field of Alzheimer's and dementia research is constantly evolving. While this book provides a snapshot of the current understanding and practices, we encourage you to stay informed about new developments. Use the resources provided to keep abreast of the latest research and advancements in care.

By engaging with this book, you are taking an important step towards enhancing the lives of those affected by Alzheimer's and dementia. We hope the information and tools provided here will offer you guidance, comfort, and the means to navigate the challenges ahead with confidence and compassion.

Chapter 1: Understanding Alzheimer's and Dementia

Greetings and welcome to the path of learning about dementia and Alzheimer's. We will go further into the complex network of memory loss in this chapter, including definitions, the science underlying it, early warning signs and symptoms, and the critical diagnostic and staging procedure. Dementia and Alzheimer's are not only illnesses; they are intricate environments that affect people all over the world—individuals, families, and communities. We equip ourselves to face the problems these disorders provide with knowledge, compassion, and resilience when we have a thorough grasp of them.

Defining Alzheimer's and Dementia

Alzheimer's disease and dementia are often used interchangeably, but they are distinct entities. Dementia is an umbrella term that encompasses a range of cognitive impairments affecting memory, thinking, and behavior.

Alzheimer's disease, on the other hand, is the most common form of dementia, comprising approximately 60-80% of cases. It is a progressive neurological disorder characterized by the buildup of abnormal proteins in the brain, leading to the gradual deterioration of cognitive function.

Checklist

Before we proceed, take a moment to reflect:

- Have you encountered anyone with Alzheimer's or dementia before?
- What do you understand about these conditions based on your previous knowledge or experiences?
- What questions or concerns do you have about Alzheimer's and dementia?

The Science of Memory Loss

Memory is a complex cognitive function that involves the encoding, storage, and retrieval of information. It relies on the intricate interplay of neurons, neurotransmitters, and brain structures such as the hippocampus and amygdala. In

Alzheimer's disease, the accumulation of beta-amyloid plaques and tau protein tangles disrupts these neural networks, impairing communication between brain cells and ultimately leading to cell death. As a result, memory loss, along with other cognitive deficits, becomes increasingly pronounced over time.

Worksheet

Consider your own experiences with memory:

- Reflect on a cherished memory from your past. What details can you recall?
- Have you ever experienced moments of forgetfulness or lapses in memory? If so, describe them.
- How do you currently maintain and strengthen your memory?

Early Signs and Symptoms

Recognizing the early signs of Alzheimer's and dementia is crucial for early intervention and effective management.

While the manifestation of symptoms may vary from person to person, common early indicators include:

1. **Memory Loss**: Forgetfulness that disrupts daily life, such as forgetting important dates or events, repeating questions, or relying on memory aids.

2. **Difficulty Performing Familiar Tasks**: Challenges with tasks that were previously routine, such as cooking, managing finances, or following instructions.

3. **Confusion and Disorientation**: Feeling lost in familiar places, becoming disoriented in time or location, or struggling to understand conversations.

4. **Changes in Mood and Behavior**: Mood swings, irritability, apathy, or withdrawal from social activities and hobbies.

5. **Trouble with Language and Communication**: Difficulty finding the right words, following conversations, or understanding written or spoken language.

Reflection Questions

Pause and reflect on the following:

- Do you recognize any of these early signs and symptoms in yourself or someone you know?
- How do these symptoms impact daily life and relationships?
- What emotions arise when considering the possibility of experiencing or witnessing these changes?

Diagnosis and Stages

Seeking a timely and accurate diagnosis is paramount in the management of Alzheimer's and dementia. While there is no single test to confirm these conditions definitively, healthcare professionals employ a comprehensive approach that includes:

1. **Medical History and Physical Examination:** Gathering information about symptoms, medical history, and medications, and conducting neurological exams to assess cognitive function.

2. **Cognitive Assessments**: Utilizing standardized tests to evaluate memory, language, attention, and other cognitive domains.

3. **Imaging Studies**: such as MRI or PET scans to detect changes in brain structure and function.

4. **Laboratory Tests**: Blood tests to rule out other potential causes of cognitive decline, such as thyroid disorders or vitamin deficiencies.

Once diagnosed, Alzheimer's and dementia are typically staged according to the progression of symptoms. While staging systems may vary, they generally include:

a. **Early Stage**: Mild cognitive impairment characterized by subtle memory lapses and occasional difficulty with tasks.

b. **Middle Stage**: Moderate decline marked by increased memory loss, confusion, and challenges with daily activities.

c. **Late Stage**: Severe cognitive impairment requiring extensive assistance with activities of daily living, loss of communication abilities, and changes in physical function.

Checklist

Take a moment to assess your understanding:

- Have you or a loved one undergone a formal evaluation for cognitive decline?
- How do you envision navigating the journey through different stages of Alzheimer's or dementia?
- What support systems and resources might be beneficial during each stage?

We have established the foundation for a more thorough understanding of dementia and Alzheimer's as we wrap up this chapter. We have started a path of knowledge and awareness, from comprehending their definitions and the underlying science of memory loss to identifying early signs and symptoms, navigating the diagnostic procedure, and staging. Equipped with understanding and compassion, we are more capable of aiding individuals impacted by these illnesses and pushing for improvements in treatment, support, and research.

Action Step

Before moving forward, take a moment to set an intention:

- How do you plan to apply the insights gained from this chapter in your personal or professional life?
- What steps will you take to deepen your understanding of Alzheimer's and dementia and support those affected by these conditions?
- Share your commitment with someone you trust to hold yourself accountable for your intentions.

Chapter 2: The Emotional Impact

Let's look at the enormous emotional impact of Alzheimer's and dementia on people who have the disease, their families, and caregivers. Beyond the physical signs, these illnesses elicit a range of emotions, from fear and loss to love and resilience. Understanding and navigating this emotional landscape is critical to developing empathy, compassion, and effective support networks.

Living with a Diagnosis

Receiving a diagnosis of Alzheimer's or dementia is a life-altering moment, both for the individual and their loved ones. It is a profound shift that encompasses a range of emotions, including shock, disbelief, anger, sadness, and uncertainty. For the person diagnosed, it may evoke feelings of loss, fear of the unknown, and a sense of vulnerability. For family members and caregivers, it often initiates a journey of mourning for the future they envisioned and adjusting to the realities of the present.

Reflection Questions

Pause and reflect on the following:

- How would you react if you or a loved one received a diagnosis of Alzheimer's or dementia?
- What emotions do you associate with the prospect of living with these conditions?
- How might your perspectives and priorities shift in response to a diagnosis?

Emotional Reactions and Support

Getting through the emotional rollercoaster of Alzheimer's and dementia involves a supporting network of family, friends, healthcare experts, and community services. Individuals and their loved ones may feel a variety of emotions along the trip, including:

1. **Grief and Loss:** Mourning the loss of cognitive abilities, independence, and future plans.

2. **Fear and Anxiety**: Anxiety about the progression of the disease, the impact on relationships, and uncertainties about the future.

3. **Frustration and Anger**: Frustration with cognitive decline, communication challenges, and changes in behavior.

4. **Love and Connection**: Finding moments of joy, connection, and intimacy amidst the challenges.

5. **Hope and Resilience**: Cultivating hope and resilience by focusing on strengths, adapting to changing circumstances, and seeking support.

Worksheet

Reflect on your support network and coping mechanisms:

- Who are the individuals or resources you turn to for emotional support?
- How do you typically cope with stress and difficult emotions?
- What self-care practices or activities bring you comfort and solace during challenging times?

The Caregiver's Role

Caregivers play a crucial role in the lives of individuals with Alzheimer's and dementia, providing physical, emotional, and practical support throughout the disease journey. However, caregiving can also be emotionally and physically taxing, leading to stress, burnout, and caregiver burden. Caregivers need to prioritize their well-being and seek support when needed.

Checklist

Assess your caregiver responsibilities and self-care practices:

- What are your primary roles and responsibilities as a caregiver?
- How do you balance caregiving duties with your own needs and obligations?
- What support systems or resources can you tap into to alleviate caregiver stress and prevent burnout?

Coping Strategies for Families

Coping with Alzheimer's and dementia as a family requires open communication, empathy, and resilience. Here are some strategies for families to navigate the emotional challenges together:

1. **Education and Information:** Educate yourselves about Alzheimer's and dementia, their progression, and available resources.

2. **Effective Communication**: Maintain open, honest, and respectful communication within the family and with the person diagnosed.

3. **Seeking Support**: Reach out to support groups, counseling services, and community organizations for emotional support and practical guidance.

4. **Establishing Routines and Boundaries**: Establish predictable routines and clear boundaries to provide stability and structure amidst uncertainty.

5. **Self-Care and Respite**: Prioritize self-care and seek respite care to prevent caregiver burnout and maintain well-being.

Action Step

Commit to implementing one coping strategy within your family:

- Which coping strategy resonates most with your family's needs and circumstances?
- How will you implement this strategy and integrate it into your daily routines?
- Share your commitment with your family members and hold each other accountable for mutual support and accountability.

As we conclude this chapter, we recognize the profound emotional impact of Alzheimer's and dementia on individuals, families, and caregivers. By acknowledging and addressing the myriad emotions accompanying these conditions, we pave the way for empathy, understanding, and resilience. Together, let us embrace the emotional journey with compassion, courage, and unwavering support.

FACT:

Alzheimer's disease and dementia are prevalent neurological disorders affecting millions worldwide. Alzheimer's disease is the most common form of dementia, accounting for approximately 60-80% of cases, while other types include vascular dementia, Lewy body dementia, and frontotemporal dementia.

Chapter 3: Medical Care and Management

Treatment Options

While there is currently no cure for Alzheimer's disease and certain forms of dementia, there are various treatment options available to manage symptoms and improve quality of life. These may include:

1. **Medications**: Drugs such as cholinesterase inhibitors (e.g., donepezil, rivastigmine) and memantine are commonly prescribed to manage cognitive symptoms and slow disease progression.

2. **Non-Pharmacological Interventions**: Therapeutic interventions such as cognitive stimulation therapy, reminiscence therapy, and music therapy can enhance cognitive function, mood, and overall well-being.

3. **Behavioral and Psychological Therapies**: Techniques such as behavioral interventions, cognitive-behavioral

therapy, and mindfulness-based approaches can help manage behavioral symptoms and improve coping skills.

4. **Lifestyle Modifications**: Adopting a healthy lifestyle that includes regular exercise, a balanced diet, social engagement, and mental stimulation can support brain health and potentially delay cognitive decline.

Reflection Questions

Pause and reflect on your understanding of treatment options:

- What treatment options have you explored or encountered in your journey with Alzheimer's or dementia?
- How do you perceive the effectiveness and challenges of pharmacological versus non-pharmacological interventions?
- What lifestyle modifications do you believe could benefit individuals living with these conditions?

Managing Daily Life

Living with Alzheimer's and dementia necessitates adapting to changes in cognitive function and daily routines. Here are some strategies for effectively managing daily life:

1. **Routine and Structure**: Establishing predictable routines and structured daily activities can provide stability and reduce anxiety.

2. **Memory Aids and Assistive Technologies**: Utilize memory aids such as calendars, reminder apps, and assistive devices to compensate for memory loss and support independence.

3. **Simplifying Tasks**: Break down complex tasks into manageable steps and provide clear, concise instructions to facilitate understanding and completion.

4. **Environmental Modifications**: Create a safe and supportive environment by removing hazards, labeling objects, and maintaining familiarity with surroundings.

5. **Empowering Independence**: Encourage and empower individuals to participate in meaningful activities and decision-making to preserve autonomy and dignity.

Checklist

Evaluate your approach to managing daily life:

- What strategies have you implemented to support daily functioning for yourself or a loved one with Alzheimer's or dementia?
- Are there any areas of daily life that present particular challenges or opportunities for improvement?
- How can you adapt your environment and routines to promote independence and well-being?

Safety Measures

Ensuring safety is paramount when caring for individuals with Alzheimer's and dementia, as they may be prone to accidents and wandering behaviors. Implementing safety measures can help mitigate risks and promote peace of mind for caregivers:

1. **Home Safety**: Modify the home environment to minimize fall hazards, secure doors and windows, and install safety locks and alarms.

2. **Identification and Communication**: Keep identification and contact information readily accessible in case of emergencies, and inform neighbors and local authorities about the individual's condition and potential wandering tendencies.

3. **Tracking Devices**: Consider using GPS tracking devices or wearable technology to monitor the individual's location and facilitate timely intervention if they wander.

4. **Medication Management**: Ensure proper medication management to prevent accidental overdoses or missed doses, and consider utilizing pill organizers or medication management apps for assistance.

5. **Emergency Preparedness**: Develop and regularly review an emergency plan with designated contacts, evacuation routes, and essential supplies in case of emergencies such as natural disasters or medical crises.

Worksheet

Create a personalized safety plan:

- Identify potential safety risks and hazards in your home environment.
- Develop strategies to address these risks and enhance safety measures.
- Share your safety plan with family members and caregivers, and review it regularly to ensure ongoing effectiveness.

Future Therapies and Research

While current treatment options focus primarily on managing symptoms, ongoing research holds promise for advancements in Alzheimer's and dementia care. Emerging therapies and research initiatives aim to target the underlying mechanisms of the disease, delay its progression, and ultimately find a cure. Some areas of active research include:

1. **Precision Medicine**: Tailoring treatment approaches based on individuals' genetic profiles and biomarkers to optimize effectiveness and minimize side effects.

2. **Immunotherapy**: Investigating the role of immune-based therapies in clearing abnormal proteins such as beta-amyloid and tau from the brain.

3. **Lifestyle Interventions**: Exploring the impact of lifestyle factors such as diet, exercise, sleep, and cognitive stimulation on brain health and disease prevention.

4. **Stem Cell Therapy**: Harnessing the regenerative potential of stem cells to repair damaged brain tissue and restore cognitive function.

5. **Genetic Editing**: Investigating gene-editing techniques such as CRISPR-Cas9 to modify or eliminate disease-causing mutations associated with Alzheimer's and dementia.

Reflection Questions

Consider the implications of future therapies and research:

- How do you envision the landscape of Alzheimer's and dementia care evolving in the future?
- What role do you see yourself playing in advocating for and participating in research initiatives?
- What hopes or concerns do you have regarding the ethical, social, and practical implications of emerging therapies?

As we conclude this chapter, we have explored the multifaceted aspects of medical care and management for Alzheimer's and dementia. From treatment options and strategies for managing daily life to safety measures and future therapies and research, we have equipped ourselves with the knowledge and resources to navigate the complexities of these conditions with diligence, compassion, and hope. As we continue on this journey, let us remain steadfast in our commitment to supporting individuals, families, and communities affected by Alzheimer's and dementia, and advocating for advancements in research, care, and support.

Action Step

Take a proactive step towards implementing one of the strategies discussed in this chapter:

- Which aspect of medical care and management resonates most with your current circumstances or interests?
- How will you integrate this strategy into your caregiving approach or personal lifestyle?
- Share your commitment with a trusted individual or support network to hold yourself accountable and seek assistance if needed.

FACT:

Diagnosis of Alzheimer's disease and dementia involves a comprehensive assessment of medical history, physical examination, cognitive testing, and brain imaging studies. While there is currently no cure for Alzheimer's disease or dementia, early diagnosis and intervention can help manage symptoms, slow disease progression, and improve quality of life through medication, cognitive therapy, and supportive care.

Chapter 4: Legal and Financial Planning

Let's look at some of the most important components of legal and financial planning for those living with Alzheimer's and dementia. As these diseases worsen, they might impair decision-making skills and money management abilities, necessitating earlier preparation to provide autonomy, protection, and peace of mind. This chapter offers complete information for managing the legal and financial complexity with foresight, care, and compassion, from planning for the future and comprehending legal papers and rights to executing financial plans and obtaining support.

Preparing for the Future

Preparing for the future involves anticipating and addressing the legal, financial, and practical implications of Alzheimer's and dementia. It is essential to plan ahead while individuals still have the capacity to make informed decisions and express their wishes. Key considerations include:

1. **Advance Directives**: Drafting advance directives such as a healthcare power of attorney and living will designate a trusted individual to make medical decisions on one's behalf and outline preferences for end-of-life care.

2. **Legal Capacity Assessment**: Assessing legal capacity with the assistance of legal and healthcare professionals to determine an individual's ability to understand and execute legal documents.

3. **Guardianship and Conservatorship**: Exploring options for guardianship or conservatorship if an individual lacks the capacity to make decisions or manage their affairs independently.

4. **Family Discussions**: Initiate open and honest discussions with family members about future plans, preferences, and responsibilities to ensure alignment and transparency.

Reflection Questions

Pause and reflect on your preparedness for the future:

- Have you taken any steps to prepare legally and financially for the possibility of Alzheimer's or dementia?
- What concerns or uncertainties do you have about planning for the future?
- How might you initiate conversations with family members about these important matters?

Legal Documents and Rights

Understanding and executing essential legal documents is crucial for protecting the rights and interests of individuals with Alzheimer's and dementia. Key documents to consider include:

1. **Wills and Trusts**: Establishing a will or trust to outline how assets and properties will be distributed upon death and designate a trusted individual to oversee estate administration.

2. **Power of Attorney**: Designating a durable power of attorney to make financial decisions and manage legal affairs on one's behalf in the event of incapacity.

3. **Healthcare Proxy**: Appointing a healthcare proxy or agent to make medical decisions and advocate for healthcare preferences when the individual is unable to do so.

4. **HIPAA Authorization**: Providing written authorization for healthcare providers to disclose protected health information to designated individuals, ensuring seamless communication and coordination of care.

Checklist

Evaluate your understanding and execution of legal documents:

- Do you have the necessary legal documents in place to protect your rights and interests in the event of incapacity?
- Have you reviewed and updated your legal documents periodically to reflect changing circumstances or preferences?
- Are there any additional legal documents or rights you wish to explore or clarify?

Financial Strategies and Assistance

Managing finances and navigating financial challenges can be particularly daunting for individuals and families affected by Alzheimer's and dementia. Here are some strategies and resources to consider:

1. **Financial Planning**: Develop a comprehensive financial plan that addresses budgeting, asset management, debt management, and long-term care funding.

2. **Long-Term Care Insurance**: Explore long-term care insurance options to help cover the costs of in-home care, assisted living, or nursing home care in the future.

3. **Government Benefits**: Determine eligibility for government benefits such as Social Security Disability Insurance (SSDI), Supplemental Security Income (SSI), and Medicaid to assist with healthcare and long-term care expenses.

4. **Elder Law Attorneys**: Consult with elder law attorneys specializing in legal issues affecting older adults, including

estate planning, Medicaid planning, and asset protection strategies.

5. **Financial Assistance Programs**: Research and access financial assistance programs offered by nonprofit organizations, community agencies, and religious institutions to provide financial support and relief for caregivers and families.

Worksheet

Create a personalized financial plan:

- Assess your current financial situation, including income, expenses, assets, and liabilities.
- Identify potential financial challenges and goals related to Alzheimer's or dementia care.
- Develop strategies and resources to address these challenges and achieve your financial goals.

In summary, we have explored the critical aspects of legal and financial planning for individuals living with Alzheimer's and dementia. By preparing for the future, understanding legal documents and rights, and implementing financial strategies and assistance, individuals and their families can navigate the complexities of these conditions with confidence and peace of mind. As we continue on this journey, let us remain proactive in addressing legal and financial considerations, advocating for the rights and dignity of those affected by Alzheimer's and dementia, and supporting each other with compassion and resilience.

Action Step

Commit to taking one concrete action towards your legal or financial planning:

- Which aspect of legal or financial planning resonates most with your current needs or concerns?
- How will you prioritize and implement this action step in your planning process?
- Share your commitment with a trusted advisor, family member, or friend to hold yourself accountable and seek support if needed.

Chapter 5: Caregiving Essentials

As Alzheimer's and dementia progress, the role of a caregiver becomes more important. It's not only about giving physical care; it's about building an environment of understanding, compassion, and support. In this chapter, we will go deep into the basics of caring, studying the fundamental factors necessary for delivering the greatest possible care for your loved one.

The Basics of Caregiving

Before getting into caring approaches, it's necessary to understand the condition itself. Alzheimer's and dementia are progressive neurological illnesses that impact memory, cognition, and behavior. Educating yourself on the phases, symptoms, and obstacles associated with these disorders helps empower you to give more effective treatment.

Caregiving for someone with Alzheimer's or dementia demands enormous patience and compassion. It's crucial to approach each conversation with empathy, realizing that the behaviors and emotions shown by your loved one are frequently beyond their control.

Communication is also crucial to giving effective treatment. However, as the condition worsens, spoken communication may become problematic. Be patient, use basic language, keep eye contact, and leverage non-verbal clues such as touch and facial expressions to deliver your message successfully.

Caring for a loved one with Alzheimer's or dementia may be emotionally and physically demanding. Remember to emphasize self-care, which includes getting enough sleep, eating well, exercising regularly, and seeking help when necessary. You can't pour from an empty cup, so taking care of oneself is critical to provide the greatest care possible.

Creating a Supportive Environment

Creating a safe atmosphere is critical for avoiding accidents and ensuring the well-being of your loved ones. Remove tripping hazards, put handrails and grab bars, use childproof locks on cabinets storing dangerous objects, and think about adding monitoring systems for extra protection.

Familiarity and comfort can significantly reduce anxiety and bewilderment in those suffering from Alzheimer's or dementia. Keep their living area neat and clutter-free, utilize familiar objects and images to trigger memories, and stick to a predictable daily schedule to create a sense of security.

Engage your loved one's senses to increase their cognitive function and enhance their general well-being. Play their favorite music, give textured things to touch, include pleasant fragrances into their surroundings, and promote taste and smell-related activities, such as cooking together.

Setting limits when giving care is critical for maintaining a successful caregiver-patient relationship. Respect your loved one's dignity and individuality, include them in decision-making whenever feasible, and establish clear boundaries to effectively handle problematic behaviors.

Daily Routine and Activities

Setting up a defined daily routine might help you and your loved one feel more stable and predictable. Create a feeling of regularity despite the turmoil of dementia by scheduling regular mealtimes, hygiene routines, medication reminders, and leisure activities.

Engage your loved one in activities that match their interests and talents. This might involve gardening, drawing, puzzles, listening to music, or looking at old photos. Adapt activities to their changing cognitive function, focusing on the process rather than the end.

Keep your loved one's mind engaged with cognitive stimulation exercises. This might include memory games, word puzzles, storytelling, or basic arithmetic activities. Tailor activities to their cognitive capacities, gradually increasing complexity as tolerated.

Encourage frequent physical activity to improve your overall health and well-being. This might include light exercises like walking, yoga, or tai chi. Exercise improves not only physical health but also mood, cognitive, and sleep quality.

Respite Care and Support Groups

Taking breaks from caring is critical for avoiding burnout and maintaining your own well-being. Consider respite care choices such as in-home caregivers, adult day programs, or short-term residential facilities. Use these resources to refuel and meet your personal needs.

Joining a support group may give vital emotional support, practical assistance, and friendship with others dealing with similar issues. Support groups, whether in person or online, provide a secure environment for people to share their experiences, vent their frustrations, and learn about caring practices.

Don't be afraid to seek expert help when necessary. Seek advice and assistance from healthcare experts, social workers, or therapists who specialize in Alzheimer's and dementia care. They can provide useful information, tailored advice, and referrals to other services as needed.

Ensure that you have legal and financial affairs in order to reduce the load and stress of caregiving. Consult an elder law attorney about establishing legal papers such as power of attorney, advance directives, and wills. Consider financial planning techniques for long-term care.

Checklist

- **Safety Checklist:** Evaluate your loved one's living environment for any safety risks and make any required changes.
- **Daily Routine Planner:** Create a daily calendar that includes meals, medicine reminders, activities, and rest intervals.
- **Activity Idea Worksheet:** Create meaningful activities based on your loved one's interests and talents.
- **Self-Care Assessment:** Evaluate your current self-care routines and identify areas for improvement.

Reflection Questions

- How has caring changed your life, both positively and negatively?
- Which tactics have you found to be the most helpful in dealing with problematic behaviors?
- How do you balance self-care with the duties of caregiving?
- Which support resources have you found most useful during your caregiving journey?

Caring for someone with Alzheimer's or dementia requires far more than just physical assistance. It demands patience, compassion, and a thorough grasp of the condition and its consequences. Create a supportive atmosphere, develop daily routines and meaningful activities, and seek respite care and assistance to improve the quality of life for both your loved one and yourself. Remember that you are not alone on this path. Seek assistance when necessary, prioritize self-care, and treasure the moments of connection and joy that occur in the middle of obstacles. Together, we can negotiate the challenges of Alzheimer's and dementia with grace and tenacity.

Chapter 6: Advance Care Considerations

As Alzheimer's and dementia worsen, caregivers frequently face complicated issues that need careful thinking and planning. In this chapter, we will be looking at advanced care alternatives including long-term care, palliative care, and end-of-life care, as well as the emotional components of grieving and loss. Caregivers can manage the disease's final phases with grace and dignity if they handle these issues with compassion and foresight.

Long-Term Care Options

Individuals with Alzheimer's or dementia can remain in their familiar surroundings while getting care from qualified caregivers. Personal care, medication administration, meal preparation, and companionship are all possible services. Examine dementia care agencies' qualifications, reputations, and suitability for your loved one's requirements.

Also, Assisted living facilities offer a supportive atmosphere for those who need help with everyday tasks but do not require round-the-clock medical care. These facilities include private or communal rooms, food, recreational activities, and help with medication administration and personal hygiene. Tour several institutions, learn about dementia care programs, and evaluate staff-to-resident ratios and safety practices.

Memory care units at assisted living facilities or nursing homes are particularly built to fulfill the requirements of people who have Alzheimer's or dementia. These complexes often have additional security, specialized programming, and dementia-trained personnel. Assess the quality of care, engagement opportunities, and resident happiness at each memory care facility you examine.

Individuals with advanced dementia or extensive medical requirements are cared for and supervised around the clock in skilled nursing facilities. These institutions provide rehabilitation, nursing, and palliative care to treat physical, cognitive, and emotional ailments. Investigate facility ratings, personnel numbers, and inspection reports to guarantee high-quality treatment and safety measures.

Palliative and End-of-Life Care

Palliative care aims to improve the quality of life for those living with severe diseases such as Alzheimer's and dementia. It treats not just bodily symptoms like pain, nausea, and difficulties breathing, but also emotional, social, and spiritual demands. Consult a palliative care team, which includes physicians, nurses, social workers, and chaplains, to create a specific care plan based on your loved one's objectives and preferences.

Hospice care offers compassionate end-of-life care to those with terminal diseases, focusing on comfort and dignity. Hospice services can be delivered at home, at a hospice facility, or in a skilled nursing facility, depending on the individual's requirements and wishes. Engage in open and honest talks with your loved one and healthcare providers about their preferences for end-of-life care, and look into hospice services in your region.

Advance care planning is discussing and documenting your loved one's preferences for medical treatment and end-of-life care while they are still able to communicate with them. This can involve decisions regarding life-sustaining therapies, resuscitation preferences, and appointing a healthcare proxy or power of attorney. Start these talks early, engage important family members and healthcare providers, and revise and update the plan as necessary.

Navigating palliative and end-of-life care may be emotionally difficult for both caregivers and loved ones. Seek help from friends, family, support groups, and mental health specialists to deal with grieving, anticipating loss, and caregiver stress. During this tough time, practice self-care practices such as mindfulness, journaling, and engaging in meaningful activities to support your emotional well-being.

Grief and Bereavement

Grief is a normal and complicated response to loss that includes a variety of feelings such as grief, anger, guilt, and desire. Recognize that mourning is a unique and personal experience impacted by elements such as the nature of the connection, the circumstances of the loss, and personal coping strategies. Allow yourself and your loved ones the time and space to grieve in their own manner, and seek help as required.

Explore healthy coping skills to help you manage the grief process effectively. This may involve freely discussing your emotions, attending support groups or therapy, participating in rituals or customs to commemorate your loved one's memory, and seeking meaning and purpose in your life going ahead. Be patient and loving with yourself as you go through the ups and downs of grieving, and allow yourself to feel joy and laughter in the middle of the pain.

Finding meaningful methods to remember your loved one can bring comfort and peace during times of mourning. Consider making a remembrance book or scrapbook with images and souvenirs, planting a tree or garden in their memory, participating in a charity walk or fundraising event, or arranging a memorial ceremony or gathering to commemorate their life and legacy.

Checklist

- **Long-Term Care Assessment:** Consider the advantages and drawbacks of several long-term care alternatives, including cost, location, amenities, and quality of care given.
- **Palliative Care Preferences:** Record your loved one's preferences for palliative care interventions, pain management techniques, and end-of-life desires.
- **Advance Directive Template:** Create an advance directive document that details your loved one's healthcare choices, treatment goals, and authorized decision-makers.
- **Grief Journal Prompts:** Use journaling prompts to reflect on your experiences with grief and bereavement, including feelings, memories, and coping mechanisms.

Reflection Questions

- What are the most essential considerations to consider when choosing long-term care for a loved one?

- How can you ensure that your loved one's final desires are recognized and honored?
- What tactics have you found useful in dealing with loss and bereavement?
- How can you help other family members or caregivers who are also grieving?

As caregivers, navigating the advanced stages of Alzheimer's and dementia necessitates careful consideration of long-term care alternatives, palliative and end-of-life decisions, and coping skills for grief and loss. Caregivers who prepare ahead of time and seek help may guarantee that their loved ones receive compassionate care while also nurturing their own emotional well-being during the caring journey. Remember that you are not alone in this journey. Even as you face the obstacles of loss and transition, rely on your support network, prioritize self-care, and appreciate the memories and moments of connection you have with your loved one.

FACT:

Alzheimer's disease and dementia result from changes in the brain, including the accumulation of abnormal protein deposits (such as beta-amyloid plaques and tau tangles), inflammation, and the loss of neurons and connections between brain cells. These changes disrupt communication between brain regions, leading to cognitive decline and memory loss.

Chapter 7: Building Awareness and Advocacy

Raising public awareness and pushing for legislative change are key components in the battle against Alzheimer's and dementia, helping to drive progress and improve the lives of individuals afflicted. This chapter will look at techniques for raising awareness, advocating for change, and gaining access to community resources and assistance. We can all work together to make the world more dementia-friendly by becoming knowledgeable and powerful advocates.

Raise Public Awareness

Educating the public about Alzheimer's and dementia is critical for debunking misunderstandings, lowering stigma, and increasing understanding and empathy. Organize educational activities, workshops, and community forums to improve awareness of dementia symptoms, risk factors, accessible services, and the disease's impact on individuals and families.

Use the power of media to raise awareness and reach a larger audience. Create targeted media campaigns that use television, radio, print, and social media channels to tell captivating tales, convey accurate information, and promote early detection and diagnosis. Collaborate with local media outlets, influencers, and advocacy groups to increase the reach and impact of your message.

Participate in or organize public events and awareness-raising campaigns to engage the community and build support for Alzheimer's and dementia activism. This might include walks, fundraisers, art shows, film screenings, or legislative lobbying days. Collaborate with neighborhood groups, companies, schools, and healthcare professionals to broaden your reach and rally support.

Advocacy and Policy Change

Advocate for policies at the local, state, and federal levels that emphasize Alzheimer's and dementia research, financing, and support services. Contact political officials, attend advocacy days, and join grassroots advocacy organizations to raise your voice and influence legislative choices. Support legislation that encourages early identification and diagnosis, broadens access to care, and strengthens caregiver support.

Encourage the development of dementia-friendly communities that are welcoming, supportive, and attentive to the needs of people living with Alzheimer's and dementia. Collaborate with local governments, companies, healthcare providers, and community groups to put dementia-friendly initiatives in place, such as first responder training, public awareness campaigns, and access to dementia-friendly activities and services.

Advocate for more financing for Alzheimer's and dementia research in order to speed up scientific discovery, expand treatment choices, and, ultimately, find a solution for these awful diseases. Support organizations and programs that prioritize research funding and engage in lobbying to keep Alzheimer's and dementia at the top of the national research agenda.

Community Resources and Support

Connect with local Alzheimer's and dementia support groups to get emotional support, practical assistance, and friendship from people going through similar experiences. Attend support group meetings in person or online, share your experiences and thoughts, and benefit from the collective expertise of other caregivers and professionals in the field.

Use helplines and hotlines manned by experienced specialists to obtain information, services, and assistance for Alzheimer's and dementia-related difficulties. These helplines offer confidential assistance, advice on caregiving practices, connections to local resources, and crisis intervention services to people and families in need.

Take advantage of respite care services to provide caregivers with short relief while ensuring that their loved ones get high-quality care during their absence. Investigate respite care choices such as in-home caregivers, adult day programs, or short-term residential facilities, and use respite vouchers or grants to help cover the cost of care.

Access online tools and digital platforms to be educated, engaged, and supported as you navigate Alzheimer's and dementia. Investigate credible websites, forums, and social media groups devoted to Alzheimer's and dementia awareness, caring advice, research updates, and community participation possibilities.

Action Plan

- **Policy Priorities Worksheet:** Determine major policy priorities and advocacy objectives for Alzheimer's and dementia awareness, research funding, and caregiver assistance.
- **Legislative Advocacy Toolkit:** Create advocacy materials like fact sheets, sample letters, and talking points to help you express your message to lawmakers.
- **Community Engagement Checklist:** Create and coordinate community events, awareness campaigns, and advocacy activities using a step-by-step checklist and timeframe.
- **Resource Directory:** Create a comprehensive list of local and national resources for Alzheimer's and

dementia education, advocacy, support groups, and helplines.

Reflection Questions

- What inspires you to promote Alzheimer's and dementia awareness and support?
- How can you use your personal experiences and talents to promote good change in your community?
- What impediments or problems do you anticipate experiencing throughout your advocacy activities, and how will you overcome them?
- What techniques can you use to maintain momentum and participation in your advocacy activity over time?

Building awareness and activism for Alzheimer's and dementia is more than a responsibility; it is a moral necessity. By promoting public awareness, lobbying for legislative reform, and gaining access to community resources and assistance, we can make a real difference in the lives of individuals impacted by these deadly diseases. Together, we can tear down barriers, combat stigma, and build a more compassionate and dementia-friendly society.

Let us continue to be change agents, advocates for progress, and beacons of hope for a better future in the battle against Alzheimer's and dementia.

FACT:

Alzheimer's disease and dementia not only affect individuals diagnosed with the condition but also have a significant impact on their caregivers and families. Caregivers often experience emotional stress, financial strain, and physical exhaustion while providing care and support for their loved ones. Access to respite care, support groups, and community resources is crucial for caregivers to maintain their own well-being while caring for someone with Alzheimer's or dementia.

Glossary of Terms

A

Activities of Daily Living (ADLs): Basic self-care tasks essential for independent living, including bathing, dressing, grooming, eating, and mobility.

Advance Directive: Legal document that outlines an individual's preferences for medical treatment and end-of-life care in the event they are unable to communicate their wishes.

Agitation: Restlessness, anxiety, or emotional distress commonly experienced by individuals with Alzheimer's or dementia.

Alzheimer's Disease: Progressive neurodegenerative disease characterized by memory loss, cognitive decline, and changes in behavior and personality.

B

Behavioral and Psychological Symptoms of Dementia (BPSD): Range of behavioral and psychological changes observed in individuals with dementia, including agitation, aggression, hallucinations, and mood disturbances.

C

Caregiver: Individual responsible for providing physical, emotional, and/or financial support to someone with Alzheimer's or dementia.

Cognition: Mental processes involved in acquiring, processing, and using information, including memory, attention, language, perception, and problem-solving.

Cognitive Decline: Progressive deterioration in cognitive function, including memory, reasoning, and judgment, often observed in individuals with Alzheimer's or dementia.

D

Dementia: Umbrella term for a group of cognitive disorders characterized by memory loss, impaired judgment, and difficulty with daily activities, resulting from damage to brain cells.

Delirium: Acute and fluctuating disturbance in attention, awareness, and cognition often caused by medical conditions, infections, or medication side effects.

Depression: Mood disorder characterized by persistent feelings of sadness, hopelessness, and loss of interest or pleasure in activities.

Diagnosis: Process of identifying a disease or condition based on symptoms, medical history, physical examination, and diagnostic tests.

E

Early-Onset Alzheimer's Disease: Form of Alzheimer's disease that develops before the age of 65, often characterized by a more rapid progression of symptoms.

End-of-Life Care: Supportive care provided to individuals with terminal illnesses, focusing on comfort, dignity, and quality of life in the final stages of life.

Executive Function: Higher-level cognitive abilities responsible for planning, organizing, problem-solving, and decision-making.

F

Frontotemporal Dementia (FTD): Type of dementia characterized by progressive degeneration of the frontal and temporal lobes of the brain, leading to changes in behavior, personality, and language.

G

Grief: Natural response to loss, encompassing a range of emotions such as sadness, anger, guilt, and longing.

Guardianship: Legal process in which a court appoints a guardian to make decisions on behalf of an individual who is deemed incapacitated or unable to make decisions for themselves.

H

Hallucination: Sensory perception of something that is not present, often experienced by individuals with dementia, such as seeing or hearing things that are not there.

Hospice Care: Supportive care provided to individuals with terminal illnesses, focusing on pain management, symptom control, and emotional support for both the patient and their family.

I

Incontinence: Loss of bladder or bowel control, common in the later stages of Alzheimer's or dementia.

In-home Care: Care provided to individuals in their own residence, often by family members or professional caregivers.

L

Long-Term Care: Comprehensive support and assistance provided to individuals who are unable to care for themselves due to chronic illness, disability, or cognitive impairment.

M

Memory Loss: Impairment or decline in the ability to remember past events, information, or experiences, commonly associated with Alzheimer's and other forms of dementia.

Mild Cognitive Impairment (MCI): Intermediate stage between normal age-related cognitive decline and dementia, characterized by noticeable memory or cognitive changes that are not severe enough to interfere significantly with daily functioning.

N

Neurodegeneration: Progressive loss of structure or function of neurons in the brain, commonly observed in neurodegenerative diseases such as Alzheimer's and Parkinson's disease.

Neurotransmitter: Chemical messenger that transmits signals between neurons in the brain, playing a crucial role in cognitive function, mood regulation, and behavior.

P

Palliative Care: Medical care focused on relieving symptoms, managing pain, and improving quality of life for individuals with serious illnesses, including Alzheimer's and dementia.

Person-Centered Care: Approach to caregiving that emphasizes the individual's preferences, needs, and values, with a focus on promoting autonomy, dignity, and quality of life.

R

Reminiscence Therapy: Therapeutic approach that involves stimulating memories and encouraging discussion about past experiences, often used to engage individuals with Alzheimer's or dementia.

Respite Care: Temporary care provided to individuals with disabilities or chronic illnesses to give their primary caregivers a break from caregiving responsibilities.

S

Sundowning: Phenomenon characterized by increased confusion, agitation, or restlessness in the late afternoon or evening, commonly experienced by individuals with dementia.

Support Group: Group of individuals who come together to share experiences, offer mutual support, and exchange information and resources related to a common issue or challenge, such as caregiving for someone with Alzheimer's or dementia.

T

Terminal Illness: Disease or condition for which there is no cure and that is expected to result in death within a relatively short period of time.

V

Validation Therapy: Therapeutic approach that involves acknowledging and validating the emotions and experiences of individuals with dementia, even if they are based on false beliefs or memories.

W

Wandering: Behavior commonly observed in individuals with dementia, characterized by aimless walking or pacing, often resulting in the person becoming lost or disoriented.

My Note

Special Bonus

Gain access to all my previous and future books

Please consider writing a review!

www.ingramcontent.com/pod-product-compliance
Lightning Source LLC
Chambersburg PA
CBHW070206230526
45471CB00002B/847